Beverly D. Baker

The Health Benefits of

Ivy Gourd

Ivy Gourd

Ivy Gourd

Table of Content

Chapter 1

Blood Sugar Control

Imagine a vine creeping through the lush greenery, bearing small, vibrant orbs of health. This is the enchanting ivy gourd, celebrated not only for its ornamental beauty but also for its remarkable health benefits, particularly in the realm of blood sugar control.

In the bustling arena of modern health concerns, the quest to manage blood sugar levels stands as a formidable challenge. Enter the humble ivy gourd, wielding its natural arsenal against the glucose spikes that threaten equilibrium. Studies have revealed its prowess in assisting individuals grappling with diabetes or those teetering on the edge of metabolic imbalance.

The secret lies within its botanical bounty. Ivy gourd, rich in bioactive compounds, operates as a gentle yet effective regulator of blood sugar. Its mechanisms of action may involve enhancing insulin sensitivity, promoting glucose uptake by cells, and inhibiting enzymes involved in carbohydrate metabolism. The result? A harmonious dance of glucose within the bloodstream, orchestrated by nature's own conductor.

But the benefits extend beyond mere glycemic control. Ivy gourd, with its low-calorie count and high fibre content, emerges as a stalwart ally in the battle against excess weight. By bestowing a feeling of satiety and nurturing digestive health, it empowers individuals on their journey towards wellness.

Picture a plate adorned with ivy gourd, its vibrant hues whispering tales of vitality and nourishment. As each tender morsel is savoured, the body receives a bounty of antioxidants – beta-carotene, lutein, and vitamin C – fortifying its defences against the ravages of oxidative stress.

In the intricate tapestry of human health, ivy gourd emerges as a thread of resilience. Its legacy spans not only blood sugar control but also encompasses realms of digestive wellness, immune fortification, and cardiovascular vitality. With each tender tendril, it weaves a narrative of holistic well-being, reminding us

Ivy Gourd

of nature's boundless bounty and its capacity to heal and

nurture.

Chapter 2

Weight Management

In the symphony of health, where every note resonates with vitality, ivy gourd emerges as a virtuoso in the realm of weight management. Picture a verdant vine winding its way through the verdant expanse, each leaf a testament to its nutritional potency, each fruit a promise of wellness.

At the heart of ivy gourd's prowess lies its dual nature: low in calories yet rich in essential nutrients. This botanical marvel serves as a beacon of balance in the tempest of modern dietary dilemmas. With each crunchy

Ivy Gourd

bite, it bestows a symphony of flavours while whispering secrets of satiety to the discerning palate.

But its charm extends beyond mere gustatory delight. Ivy gourd, with its generous bounty of dietary fibre, becomes a stalwart companion in the quest for a trimmer silhouette. As it traverses the digestive tract, fibre weaves a tapestry of fullness, gently urging moderation and restraint. The result? A harmonious dance of appetite and satisfaction, guided by the gentle hand of nature.

Yet, ivy gourd's contribution to weight management transcends the confines of calorie counting. Within its emerald embrace lie a plethora of vitamins, minerals, and antioxidants — a veritable cornucopia of nourishment. With each tender tendril, it bestows a bounty of beta-carotene, vitamin C, and lutein, fortifying the body against the onslaught of oxidative stress and inflammation.

Imagine a plate adorned with ivy gourd, its vibrant hues a testament to nature's artistry, its flavours a celebration of culinary ingenuity. As each delectable morsel is savoured, the body receives a treasure trove of nutrients – a feast for the senses and a boon for wellness.

In the grand tapestry of human health, ivy gourd emerges as a beacon of balance and vitality. Its legacy, woven with the threads of nutrition and flavour, serves as a reminder of nature's boundless bounty and its capacity to nourish both body and soul.

Chapter 3

Rich in Antioxidants

In the enchanting world of botanical wonders, ivy gourd stands as a beacon of vibrancy and vitality, its verdant tendrils weaving tales of resilience and renewal. Amidst the lush foliage, this humble vine bears treasures beyond compare – a symphony of antioxidants that dazzle the senses and invigorate the soul.

Picture a sun-kissed morning, dewdrops glistening like diamonds upon the emerald leaves of ivy gourd. Within each delicate orb lies a secret of nature's alchemy – a potent cocktail of beta-carotene, lutein, and vitamin C, awaiting discovery by the discerning palate.

Ivy Gourd

But what sets ivy gourd apart is not merely its ornamental beauty, but rather its profound impact on human health. As these antioxidants grace the body with their presence, they embark on a noble quest to vanquish the scourge of free radicals – those insidious agents of ageing and disease.

Beta-carotene, with its golden hue, serves as a shield against the ravages of oxidative stress, protecting delicate cells from premature ageing and degeneration. Lutein, with its radiant glow, bestows upon the eyes a mantle of protection, guarding against the onset of age-related macular degeneration.

And then there is vitamin C, the undisputed champion of immune fortification and collagen synthesis. With each succulent bite of ivy gourd, the body receives a bounty of this vital nutrient, empowering it to withstand the onslaught of infections and ailments.

But the benefits extend far beyond mere physical health. In the realm of holistic wellness, ivy gourd emerges as a muse for the soul, its vibrant hues and invigorating flavours a source of joy and inspiration. With each tender tendril, it whispers tales of resilience and renewal, reminding us of nature's boundless bounty and its capacity to nourish both body and spirit.

So, as you savour the delicate essence of ivy gourd, remember that you are not merely partaking in a culinary

Ivy Gourd

delight, but embarking on a journey of rejuvenation and vitality. Let each delectable morsel be a tribute to the splendour of nature and the enduring beauty of the human spirit.

Chapter 4

Improves Digestive Health

Journey into the verdant depths of wellness, where the ivy gourd reigns supreme as a guardian of digestive vitality. Picture a lush garden, alive with the vibrant hues of this botanical marvel, each tender leaf and plump fruit a testament to its nurturing embrace.

At the core of ivy gourd's charm lies its affinity for the intricate dance of digestion. With each delectable bite, it bestows upon the body a veritable treasure trove of dietary fibre – nature's gentle broom, sweeping away the detritus of modern living and ushering in a renewed sense of balance and harmony.

Ivy Gourd

But its magic transcends mere mechanical action. Within the emerald embrace of the ivy gourd lie a host of bioactive compounds, each with a unique role to play in the symphony of digestion. From enzymes that aid in nutrient absorption to phytonutrients that soothe inflamed tissues, this botanical wonder serves as a beacon of healing and renewal.

Imagine a table adorned with ivy gourd, its verdant hues a feast for the eyes and its flavours a symphony for the senses. As each succulent morsel is savoured, the body receives a gentle caress of nourishment – a reminder of nature's boundless bounty and its capacity to heal and nurture.

Ivy Gourd

But the benefits extend beyond mere digestive ease. In the grand tapestry of human health, ivy gourd emerges as a stalwart ally in the quest for overall wellness. Its legacy, woven with the threads of fibre and phytonutrients, serves as a reminder of the intimate connection between gut health and vitality.

So, as you embark on your journey towards digestive vitality, remember the humble ivy gourd – a botanical marvel that offers not only sustenance for the body but also solace for the soul. With each tender tendril, it whispers tales of renewal and rejuvenation, inviting you to embrace the abundant gifts of nature and reclaim your rightful place in the circle of wellness.

Chapter 5

Boosts Immune Function

In the ever-evolving saga of human health, where battles are fought against invisible adversaries, ivy gourd emerges as a valiant defender of the body's fortress – the immune system. Picture a verdant vine, weaving its way through the tapestry of life, each delicate tendril a testament to nature's resilience and ingenuity.

At the heart of ivy gourd's charm lies its bounty of bioactive compounds, each with a unique ability to bolster the body's defences against invading pathogens. As these botanical warriors course through the bloodstream, they engage in a noble quest to fortify the immune response, ensuring that the body remains steadfast in the face of adversity.

But the magic of the ivy gourd extends beyond mere fortification. Within its emerald embrace lie a plethora of vitamins and minerals, each playing a vital role in the symphony of immunity. From vitamin C, the undisputed champion of immune function, to zinc, the silent sentinel guarding against infection, this botanical wonder offers a cornucopia of nourishment for the body's defenders.

Imagine a table adorned with ivy gourd, its vibrant hues a testament to nature's bounty and its flavours a celebration of culinary ingenuity. As each succulent morsel is savoured, the body receives a veritable feast of

Ivy Gourd

immune-boosting nutrients – a shield against the onslaught of infections and ailments.

But the benefits of ivy gourd transcend the physical realm. In the grand tapestry of human health, it emerges as a beacon of resilience and vitality, reminding us of the intimate connection between body and soul. With each tender tendril, it whispers tales of renewal and rejuvenation, inviting us to embrace the abundant gifts of nature and reclaim our rightful place in the circle of wellness.

So, as you partake in the delicate essence of an ivy gourd, remember that you are not merely nourishing the body, but also nurturing the spirit. Let each delectable

bite be a tribute to the splendour of nature and the enduring resilience of the human spirit.

bite be a tribute to the splendour of nature and the

Chapter 6

Anti-inflammatory Properties

Enter the enchanted realm of botanical marvels, where the ivy gourd reigns supreme as a healer and guardian of wellness. Picture a verdant landscape, alive with the vibrant hues of this humble vine, each delicate tendril a whisper of nature's wisdom and grace.

At the heart of ivy gourd's magic lies its potent arsenal of bioactive compounds, each imbued with the power to soothe inflamed tissues and quell the fires of inflammation. As these botanical warriors traverse the pathways of the body, they engage in a noble quest to restore balance and harmony to the delicate dance of immunity and inflammation.

But the charm of the ivy gourd extends beyond mere physiological action. Within its emerald embrace lies a sanctuary for the weary soul, a refuge from the storms of modern living. With each tender tendril, it offers solace and healing, inviting us to surrender to the gentle embrace of nature's embrace.

Imagine a table adorned with ivy gourd, its vibrant hues a feast for the eyes and its flavours a symphony for the senses. As each succulent morsel is savoured, the body receives a balm of nourishment – a reminder of nature's boundless bounty and its capacity to heal and nurture.

Ivy Gourd

But the benefits of ivy gourd transcend the confines of the physical realm. In the grand tapestry of human health, it emerges as a beacon of resilience and vitality, reminding us of the intimate connection between body and soul. With each tender tendril, it whispers tales of renewal and rejuvenation, inviting us to embrace the abundant gifts of nature and reclaim our rightful place in the circle of wellness.

So, as you partake in the delicate essence of an ivy gourd, remember that you are not merely nourishing the body, but also nourishing the spirit. Let each delectable bite be a tribute to the splendour of nature and the enduring beauty of the human spirit.

Chapter 7

Supports Heart Health

In the symphony of life, where each beat echoes with vitality, ivy gourd emerges as a guardian of the body's most vital organ – the heart. Picture a lush garden, alive with the vibrant hues of this botanical marvel, each tender tendril a testament to nature's boundless bounty and its capacity to nurture and heal.

At the core of ivy gourd's charm lies its bounty of nutrients, each playing a vital role in the intricate dance of cardiovascular wellness. From potassium, the silent conductor orchestrating fluid balance and blood pressure regulation, to fibre, the gentle broom sweeping away the

Ivy Gourd

detritus of modern living, this botanical wonder offers a symphony of nourishment for the heart and soul.

But the magic of the ivy gourd extends beyond mere physiological action. Within its emerald embrace lies a sanctuary for the weary spirit, a refuge from the storms of daily life. With each tender tendril, it offers solace and healing, inviting us to surrender to the gentle rhythm of nature's embrace.

Imagine a table adorned with ivy gourd, its vibrant hues a feast for the eyes and its flavours a celebration of culinary ingenuity. As each succulent morsel is savoured, the body receives a bounty of heart-healthy nutrients – a shield against the ravages of cardiovascular disease and a testament to the power of nature's healing touch.

But the benefits of ivy gourd transcend the confines of the physical realm. In the grand tapestry of human health, it emerges as a beacon of resilience and vitality, reminding us of the intimate connection between body and soul. With each tender tendril, it whispers tales of renewal and rejuvenation, inviting us to embrace the abundant gifts of nature and reclaim our rightful place in the circle of wellness.

So, as you partake in the delicate essence of an ivy gourd, remember that you are not merely nourishing the body, but also nurturing the spirit. Let each delectable

Ivy Gourd

bite be a tribute to the splendour of nature and the
enduring beauty of the human spirit.

Chapter 8

Nutrient-Rich

Step into the lush tapestry of nature's bounty, where the ivy gourd reigns as a treasure trove of vital nutrients, each delicate tendril a testament to the abundance of life. Picture a verdant garden, alive with the vibrant hues of this botanical marvel, each tender leaf and plump fruit a celebration of nourishment and vitality.

At the heart of ivy gourd's charm lies its rich array of vitamins and minerals, each playing a vital role in the symphony of human health. From vitamin A, the guardian of vision and cellular integrity, to vitamin C, the undisputed champion of immune function and

Ivy Gourd

collagen synthesis, this botanical wonder offers a veritable cornucopia of nourishment for the body and soul.

But the magic of the ivy gourd extends beyond mere physiological action. Within its emerald embrace lies a sanctuary for the weary spirit, a refuge from the chaos of modern living. With each succulent bite, it offers solace and healing, inviting us to surrender to the gentle rhythm of nature's embrace.

Imagine a table adorned with ivy gourd, its vibrant hues a feast for the eyes and its flavours a symphony for the senses. As each delectable morsel is savoured, the body receives a bounty of essential nutrients – a shield against the ravages of deficiency and a testament to the power of nature's healing touch.

But the benefits of ivy gourd transcend the confines of the physical realm. In the grand tapestry of human health, it emerges as a beacon of resilience and vitality, reminding us of the intimate connection between body and soul. With each tender tendril, it whispers tales of renewal and rejuvenation, inviting us to embrace the abundant gifts of nature and reclaim our rightful place in the circle of wellness.

So, as you partake in the delicate essence of an ivy gourd, remember that you are not merely nourishing the body, but also nurturing the spirit. Let each delectable

Ivy Gourd

bite be a tribute to the splendour of nature and the enduring beauty of the human spirit.